5
Wealth
Architecture

DESIGNING YOUR PATH TO FINANCIAL GREATNESS"

DIXIT DHANANI

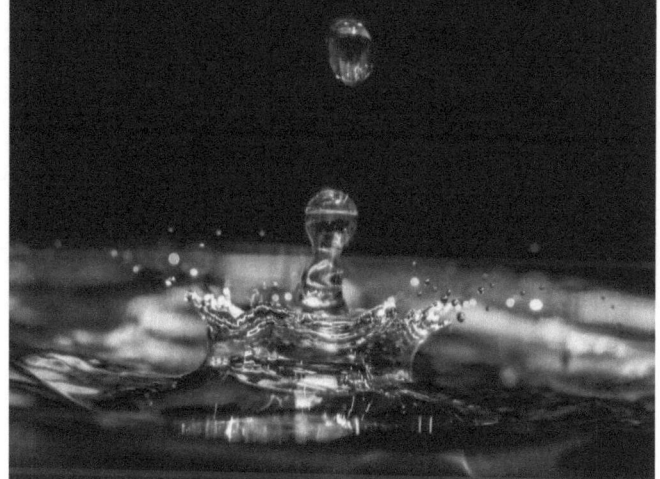

First Edition:- 2022

Second Edition:- 2023

Publisher by:- Amazon Kindle Publisher

Editor by:- Dixit Dhanani

Dedication

I will use my book to target youngsters and teach them how to increase their wealth by using the best path, which will lead to my ultimate goal of helping people to be financially free at the age of 40.

Acknowledgement

I am thankful to mr. som bathla and inspiring jatin who encourage me to write the book and help me to find the niches. That helps me to share my knowledge with society, especially to the youngsters.

I also, thanks to my parents, make me strong enough that I can launch my book at the age of 20. They always support me in every situation and give me motivation to serve the society.

I also thanks to my friend who help me in the promotion of my book "The wealth Architecture"

Contents

Chapter **-1** What is a systematic investment plan(sip)... 11

Chapter - **2** Where Your Money Invested in SIP.. 26

Chapter - 3 Mutual Fund... 33

Chapter - 4 stories.. 44

Chapter - 5 MMS technique.. 58

Chapter - 6 Is Something Better Than a Mutual Fund?.. 71

Chapter - 7 Credit Card... 83

Chapter -1

What is systematic investment plan (sip)

A Systematic investment plan more popularly as sip is a facility offered by mutual funds to the investment to invest in a disciplined manner. SIP facility allows an investor to invest in the selected mutual fund scheme or by itself. The fixed amount of money invested in the market, while the pre-defined SIP invested can be on a weekly/monthly/quarterly/semi-annually, or annual basis. By taking the sip route to investments, the investor invests in a time-bound manner without worrying about the market dynamics and stands to benefit in the long term due to average costing and the power of compounding.

Now the question is what is the power of compounding?

The power of compounding can be compared to the snowball effect, where a small ball of snow grows larger as it rolls down the slope

In the same way, compounding helps in increasing your savings by accumulating more returns on the interest earned on the initial principal investment. compounding essentially earns 'interest on interest', which means you will not only earn the interest on your initial saving but also earn additional interest at this stage.

Eventually, compounding interest helps in building wealth over the years.

For example, suppose you have received 1 lakh as an incentive and want to invest it in mutual funds. If you invest the entire 1 lakh on a single day, then you have made a Lum sum investment. On the other hand, if you decide to invest this 1 lakh Over for a 10-month period, then you have done a SIP of 10000.

Now, this does not mean that you have to log in to your bank account every month and manually transfer 10000 on the same date every time. SIPs are automated, which means that you only have to register once. Thereafter, it is automatically debited from your account and invested in the mutual fund schemes. You are free to select the SIP date and the SIP frequency- daily, weekly, monthly or quarterly.

How Does a SIP Work?

When you register a SIP, you are using your capital to buy units of mutual fund schemes or shares but we took the example of a mutual fund. These units are sold to you on a net assets value (NAV). Think of NAV as the purchase price of any goods and series. If you pay Rs 10 for a pen, then the pen's NAV is Rs 10. Similarly, mutual funds units are also bought and sold based on NAV. An important thing to note here is that NAV remains the same for Lum sum and SIP.

Now assume I want to start a SIP of RS 5000 in a Canara Rebeca blue-chip equity Fund. The fund's NAV i.e. The price of one unit of the funds is Rs 41.88. So, the funds will allot me 119.38 units. (Rs 5000/Rs 41.88). Now, if the NAV of the fund on 30th Sep 2022 is RS 42.88, then I will get 116.6 units. This brings us to an interesting observation-

· When NAV goes up = your SIP fetches fewer units.

· When NAV falls = your SIP will fetch more units.

The NAV of a mutual fund scheme is never constant. It goes up and down as per the market. Now you might think that in that case, NAV should never go up or should be constant. This way you will get more units. But you will miss out on the biggest advantage of SIP- **Rupee Cost Averaging.**

Benefits of a SIP

1.   Rupee-cost-averaging: This is one of the biggest advantages of SIP. Rupee cost against market ups and down. It averages your purchase cost and maximises returns. Suppose an investor starts a sip of Rs 500 per month for 12 months. This is how rupee cost averaging will work for him.

·   The NAV in January is Rs 15, so he will get 33.33 units (500/15).

·   The NAV in March falls to 10. Now, he will get the 50 units (500/10).

This keeps on happening throughout the year. At the end of the 12 months, he accumulated 484 units at an average cost of Rs 12.67 per unit. Now suppose he had selected to invest the entire 6000 (Rs 500*12) in January itself. He would accumulate 400 units at an average of Rs 15 per unit.

So, rupee cost averaging has helped him accumulate more units (484 vs 400) at a lower cost (12.67 vs 15). Rupees cost averaging helps you get more units when the markets are lagging and fewer units when markets are booming.

2. **Power of Compounding**: The second biggest advantage of a SIP is that it manifests the power of compounding. That we discussed earlier. The concept of compounding interest is that interest is added back to the principal amount. So,

SIP	ROR	time Frame	Future values
1000	15%	20 Year	7.59 lakh
2000	15%	20 Year	15.18 lakh
5000	15%	20 Year	49.96 lakh
10,000	15%	20 Year	99.91 lakh

interest is a compounding period. Due to this, a small sum of money regularly can grow into a huge corpus. Like a small snowball rolling.

If you start a sip of Rs 1,000 every month for the next 20 years, then you have to invest a total of Rs 2.4 lakhs only. Now due to the power of compounding, your corpus is worth a whopping Rs 7.59 lakhs. It's almost 3x your money.

3. Long-term wealth creation: The best aspect of the SIP is that investors can start with as little as Rs 100 and still build a decent-sized corpus. However humongous your corpus will be. The graph shows wealth creation by starting SIP at various stages in life.

Regular investments done with a long holding period bring benefits of compounding. The table below connotes the retirement corpus of four individuals who start investing Rs 1000 per month at 20, 30, 40 and 50 years of age in an equity fund offering 12% per year

Age at which individual starts investment	Amount Invested	Retirement Corpus
20 Years	Rs 4.8 lakh	Rs 97.93 lakh
30 Years	Rs 3.6 lakh	Rs 30.80 lakh
40 Years	Rs 2.4 lakh	Rs 9.19 lakh
50 Years	Rs 1.2 lakh	Rs 2.24 lakh

Note: Retirement age is assumed to be 60 years

As you can see, a SIP of Rs 5000 for 20 years can help you to create a corpus of Rs 75.79 lakhs. But if you just add another 5 years or 3 lakhs, your money grows from 75 lakhs to Rs 1.64 crores! Hence, if you want a huge corpus then you must start investing early and stay invested for the long team.

If you believe that starting late can be compensated by investing more, then you are in for a surprise. Otis starts a SIP of Rs 5000 for 20 years. His corpus at the end of 20 years is 75.79 lakhs. While Martin doubles his SIP amount to Rs 10,000 but still the corpus was only Rs 67.68 lakhs. Hence, SIP helps in creating long-term wealth only if you give it ample time.

	Time frame	SIP	future value
Otis	20 years	Rs 5000	Rs 75,79,774
Martin	15 years	Rs 10,000	Rs 67,68,630

4. **Disciplined approach:** The majority of investors miss out on the benefits of SIP because they are obsessed with timing the market. However, truth be told, there is no guaranteed way of predicting market movements. And by delaying your investments, you are missing out on one of the most precious resources, time. SIP helps inculcate investment discipline in investors who do not have stress in trying to time the market. Simply continue your SIPs, especially when the market is down, and reap the power of compounding.

5. **Simple, Convenient & Affordable:** SIP is highly convenient. it authorises your bank to make hassle-free payments without your involvement every single time. So, once a SIP is registered, all future payment is automatically debited from your account without your supervision. Another key advantage of SIP is that it is highly affordable. Investors can start SIP with as little as Rs 100.

6. **Higher Inflation-Adjusted Return:** If you are a small-time investor and do not possess the resources to play with the big-league players, then SIP is the solution. With SIP, even retail investors can earn above-average inflation-

beating returns compared to traditional instruments like recurring deposits, fixed deposits, and PPFs. The diversified portfolio of the scheme.

7. **Acts as an Emergency fund:** Being an open-ended fund without any tenor, you can without your SIP investment as a contingent fund. It also helps at the time of retirement. After the maturity of the scheme Lum-sum amount of the corpus is credited to your account.

Types of SIP

There are a total of 7 types of SIPS. And I will tell you which systematic investment plans are the best to invest in. And which type of SIP you select.

1. **Regular SIP**

A regular SIP is the simplest type of investment plan. Under this SIP, the investor invests a fixed amount at regular intervals. The SIP frequency can be preferred on a monthly basis. While choosing the SIP, investors can mention the SIP duration, instalment amount, and frequency. In a regular SIP, one cannot change the investment amount during the tenure of the investment.

2. **Top-up SIP**

Top-up SIP or step-up SIP allows investors to increase their SIP amount periodically. Many asset management companies have a provision to step-up SIPs. Choosing step-up SIP adds more flexibility to the recurring contributions and helps investors in parking bigger amounts. This will help them create their investment corpus faster because of the power of compounding. Therefore, it is advisable to choose SIP plans that offer this facility to top up the investments.

Furthermore, one can step up their SIP plans in multiples of INR 500. For example, if an investor is investing INR 10,000 in a mutual fund scheme and opts for a step-up every year by INR 1,000. The SIP amount from the 13th month onwards will become INR 11,000. A regular top-up of the mutual fund investments will enable investors to generate their investment corpus sooner. Moreover, it also helps in reducing the effects of inflation on the maturity corpus.

3. Flexible SIP

As the name suggests, a flexible SIP gives its investors the opportunity to alter their investment amount. It is also known as Flexi SIP or Flex SIP. One can intimate the fund house of the changes in the SIP amount or contributions. However, the intimation has to be given at least a week before the deduction date of the SIP instalment. Investors can adjust their SIP amount based on their financial conditions or market conditions. For market conditions, there is a pre-decided formula that allows investors to invest more when the markets are falling and reduce the SIP amount when the markets are high.

For example, if an investor is facing a cash crunch, they can inform the fund house to halt their SIP payments until further notice. This allows investors to skip their SIP instalments without defaulting. Similarly, if an investor has surplus cash, they can increase their SIP amount for a certain duration. Therefore, as per the investor's instructions, the fund house will be able to adjust the SIP amounts.

4. Perpetual SIP

While filling out the SIP application form, the investor has to select the tenure of the SIP. If no tenure is specified, then the SIP becomes a perpetual SIP. In other words, the SIP will continue for a duration until the investor provides instructions to the fund house or the manager to stop the investments. Also, in case an investor doesn't wish to limit their contributions with a maturity tenure, they can voluntarily choose the perpetual SIP option in the application form. This allows the investor to stay invested for longer durations and observe the market. And, in the future, they can decide to redeem at any time.

5. Trigger SIP

Trigger SIP is suitable only for those investors who are well aware of the market dynamics and are sure of its movements. In this type of systematic investment plan, it is very important to know when to take the buy and sell positions. Under this type of SIP, investors can set their SIP start date or redeem or switch their SIP once the selected event occurs. The trigger can be set to any event. For example, a favourable market event, or an index level or NAV of the fund, or capital appreciation or depreciation. Also, it is important to note that the triggering SIP is recommended only for experienced investors as it incites speculations. It is essential to have sound knowledge and experience to set appropriate triggers effectively

6. SIP With Insurance

A few asset management companies offer insurance coverage if an investor opts for long-duration investments. The initial cover for the insurance is usually ten times the first SIP amount, and it gradually increases with time. Also, this feature is available only for equity mutual funds. It is important to note that term insurance is just an add-on feature and doesn't have any impact on the performance of the fund.

7. Multi SIP

A multi-SIP allows investors to start investing in multiple schemes of a fund house through a single instrument. This helps investors in diversifying their investment portfolio. Furthermore, it also reduces the number of paperwork. Investors can give a single form and payment instructions to start their SIP plans.

Which type of systematic investment plan is best to invest?

From the above seven types of SIPS, which one is the best sip? That depends on the investor's goals, income, and knowledge. A regular SIP best suits all kinds of investors who have a regular source of income and who prefer saving up for a secured future. A step-up SIP helps reach the financial goal faster and helps in accumulating a higher amount of corpus as the investment keeps increasing every year. A perpetual SIP is a regular SIP that continues till eternity. It can be both regular as well as step-up SIP.

Flexible SIP is suitable for people with varying income levels, for example, professionals and freelancers. Trigger SIP only suits investors who have knowledge about market dynamics. SIP with insurance is a new type of plan, and investors hardly have options available in the market. Investors should opt only for this type of plan if the fund performance is good, and the life cover provided by the fund house is free.

Multi SIP only works when all the mutual funds of a fund house are giving good returns in their category.

SIP is an investment plan that allows investors to invest regularly. Through SIP, one has to invest the same amount regularly or increase the amount of SIP due to market dynamics or having additional income at hand. Therefore, we will compare a regular SIP and a step-up SIP and see which one gives better returns over some time

Example

An investor wants to accumulate a corpus of INR 25 lakhs in 10 years. He has the option to invest in a regular SIP and a top-up SIP. Let's see the returns and SIP amount needed in the case of a regular SIP and a step-up SIP. Let us assume he tops up his SIP by 10% each year.

Regular SIP

Investment: INR 5,000 a month

Tenure: 10 years or 120 months

Total investment: INR 6,00,000

Expected return: 12% per annum

Expected maturity corpus: INR 11,61,695

Return: INR 5,61,695

Step-up SIP

Investment: INR 5,000 a month

Tenure: 10 years or 120 months

Total investment: INR 9,56,148

Expected return: 12% per annum

Expected maturity corpus: INR 16,87,163

Return: INR 7,31,015

The returns from top-up SIP are higher than regular SIP for investing for the same tenure. If the investor wants to accumulate a corpus of 11.61 lakhs by doing a regular SIP, it would take ten years. But in the case of step-up SIP, the investor can reach the target of INR 11.61 lakhs in 8 years. Hence a step-up SIP is the best as it not only allows investors to reach the target amount faster but also allows investors to combat the effects of inflation. As the purchasing power reduces with a rise in inflation, a higher maturity corpus will increase the investment's real return.

What type of SIP Should Select

Investors should select a SIP type that best suits their financial requirements, knowledge, and goals. A regular SIP allows investors to invest in a SIP regularly without a pause or top-up. A step-up SIP will increase the investment amount of SIP every year. Perpetual SIP is a SIP till eternity. Investors with regular income can invest in all these SIPs.

A Flex SIP best suits investors with irregular income. Freelancers, professionals, and people with no job safety can consider investing in this SIP as they have the freedom to increase, decrease, pause and restart the SIP as per their wish.

A Trigger SIP best suits an investor who understands the market and its dynamics. An investor who doesn't understand investing or how the market works shouldn't pick a trigger SIP.

A Multi SIP allows investors to invest in different funds of a fund house. But not all the funds of a fund house tend to perform well. Hence investors have to practise caution while selecting this type of systematic investment plan.

Chapter - 2

Where Your Money Invested in SIP

Your invested money can be utilised in three types of markets those are: -

1. Equity market

2. Debt market and

3. Money market.

The equity market is consisting of

1. Share and

2. Equity-related securities

The Debt Market are consisting of

1. Government Securities

2. Bonds

3. Debentures

4. Treasury Bill

5. Commercial papers

Money Market are consisting of

1. Call and

2. Repurchase Agreement (REPO)

What is the Equity Market?

Equity markets are the meeting point for buyers and sellers of stocks. The securities traded in the equity market can either be public stocks, which are those listed on the stock exchange or privately traded stocks. Often, private stocks are traded through dealers, which is the definition of the over-the-counter market.

When companies are born, they are private companies, after a certain time, they go through an initial public offering (IPO), which is a process that turns them into public companies traded on a stock exchange. Private stocks operate slightly differently as they are only offered to employees and certain investors.

Some of the largest equity markets, or stock markets, in the world are the New York Stock Exchange, Nasdaq, Tokyo Stock Exchange, Shanghai Stock Exchange, and Nifty-50

What is the Debt market?

Debt security investments generally have lower returns in comparison to equities. However, since debt investments do not fluctuate as much as stocks, the risk involved is also much less.

Moreover, in the event that a company has to be liquidated, the business' bondholders are paid first.

The most common debt instrument is a bond. Bonds are issued by the government and corporations to raise funds for their undertakings and business operations. The interest rates for these investments tend to be fixed, and while they may be unsecured, third-party agents attest to the integrity and legitimacy of the bond issuer in the form of ratings.

Treasury bill-

Treasury Bills (T-Bills) are investment vehicles that allow investors to lend money to the government. In return, the investors get a steady interest income. The maturity period for a treasury bill is less than one year.

Commercial papers-

Companies generally use commercial papers to fund their short-term working capital needs, such as payment of accounts receivable, inventory purchases, etc. However, these are unsecured in nature

Bonds-

Borrowers issue bonds to raise money from investors willing to lend them money for a certain amount of time. When you buy a bond, you are lending to the issuer, which may be a government, municipality, or corporation

Government securities-

Government securities are debt instruments of a sovereign government. They sell these products to finance day-to-day governmental operations and provide funding for special infrastructure and military projects. These investments work in much the same way as a corporate debt issue.

Debentures: -

A debenture is a type of bond or another debt instrument that is unsecured by collateral. Since debentures have no collateral backing, they must rely on the creditworthiness and reputation of the issuer for support.

What is the Money Market?

The money market basically refers to a section of the financial market where financial instruments with high liquidity and short-term maturities are traded. The money market has become a component of the financial market for buying and selling securities of short-term maturities, of one year or less.

Over-the-counter trading is done in the money market, and it is a wholesale process. It is used by the participants as a way of borrowing and lending for the short term.

The money market consists of negotiable instruments. and certificates of deposit. It is used by many participants, including companies, to raise funds by selling commercial papers in the market. The money market is considered a safe place to invest due to the high liquidity of securities.

It has certain risks that investors should be aware of, one of them being default on securities such as commercial papers. The money market consists of various financial institutions and dealers, who seek to borrow or loan securities. It is the best source to invest in liquid assets.

The money market is an unregulated and informal market and not structured like the capital markets, where things are organised in a formal way. The money market gives lesser returns to investors who invest in it but provides a variety of products.

Withdrawing money from the money market is easier. Money markets are different from capital markets as they are for a shorter period of time while capital markets are used for longer periods.

Meanwhile, a mortgage lender can create protection against a fallout risk by entering an agreement with an agency or private conduit for operational, rather than mandatory, delivery of the mortgage. In such an agreement, the mortgage originator effectively buys an option, which gives the lender the right, but not the obligation, to deliver the mortgage. Against that, the private conduit charges a fee for allowing optional delivery.

Call money: -

Call money is one of the most liquid instruments. The validity is generally one working day. Banks can face shortfalls that can be solved by borrowing through call money. In contrast, those with surplus cash can invest in other banks through call money.

REPO: -

Repo is a repurchase agreement with repo as its abbreviation. For example, Bank A is in need of funds, while Bank B has surplus funds. Bank A will enter into an agreement with Bank B to sell its securities. Bank B will receive the required funds. However, on a fixed date in the future, Bank A will repurchase these securities from Bank B as part of the agreement.

Chapter - 3

Mutual Fund

Over the long-term horizon, equity investment has given returns that far exceed those of the debt-based instrument. They are probably the only investment option, which can build large wealth. In the short term, equity exhibits very sharp volatilizes, which many of us find difficult to stomach. Investment in equity requires one to be in constant touch with the market and do a lot of research.

Buying good scripts requires one to invest fairly large amounts. Systematic investment in a mutual fund is the answer to preventing the pitfalls of equity investment and still enjoying a high return. And it makes all the more sense today when the stock market is booming.

Management of the fund by professionals or experts is one of the key advantages of investing through a mutual fund. They regularly carry out extensive research – on the company, the industry, and the economy - thus ensuring informed investment. Secondly, they regularly track the market.

Thus, for many of us who do not desire expertise and are too busy with our vocation to devote sufficient time and effort to invest in equity, a mutual fund offers an attractive alternative. Another advantage of investment through a mutual fund is that even with a small amount we are able to enjoy the benefits of diversification. A huge amount would be required for an individual to achieve the desired diversification, which would not be possible for many of us. Diversification reduces the overall impact on the return from a portfolio, on account of loss in a particular company/sector. The mutual fund industry is well-regulated in both SEBI and AMFI. They have, over the years, introduced regulations, which ensure the smooth and transparent functioning of the mutual fund industry. This makes it safe and convenient for investors to invest through mutual funds.

One of the biggest difficulties in equity investing is WHEN to invest, apart from the other big question of WHERE to invest. While investing in a mutual fund solves the issues of 'where' to invest, SIP helps us to overcome the problems of 'when'. SIP is a discipline of investing irrespective of the state of the market. It thus makes the market timing irrelevant.

With the next 2-3 years looking good from any country's economic point of view, especially a developed country, one can expect handsome returns through regular investing. The mutual fund makes investment easier as it does not strain our income. It, therefore, becomes an ideal investment option for a small-time investor, who would otherwise not be able to enjoy the benefit of investing in the equity market.

In SIP we are investing a fixed amount regularly. Therefore, we and up buying a greater number of units when the market is down, and the NAV is low and less number of units when the market is up and the NAV is high. Generally, we would stay away from buying when the markets are down. We generally tend to invest when the markets are rising. SIP works as a good discipline as it forces us to buy even when the market is low, which actually is the best time to buy.

Mutual funds are investment companies that pool money from investors at large and offer to sell and back their shares on a continuous basis and use the capital thus raised in securities of different companies. In this, your amount is invested in different companies according to percentage ratio. A mutual fund is not an alternative investment option to stock and bond; rather it pools the money of several investors and invests this in stocks, bonds, money market instruments, and other types of securities.

A mutual fund is a trust that pools the savings of a number of investors who share a common financial goal. The money thus collected is then invested in a capital market instrument such as shares, debentures, and other securities. The income earned through these investments and the capital appreciation realised is shared by its unit holders in proportion to the number of units owned by them. Thus, a Mutual fund is the most suitable investment for the common man as it offers an opportunity to invest in a diversified, professionally managed basket of securities at a relatively low cost.

Advantages

- It is very difficult for many individuals to manage their own money. It is tough to study and analyse companies and transact to buy /sell different securities on one's own. A mutual fund gives you a professional fund manager for a small fee. This fund manager buys or sells companies, analyses them, and tracks them regularly.

- Secondly, mutual funds help you diversify your investments. When you invest only in a single security, you could risk a loss if the market crashes. However, you can avoid this problem by investing in different asset classes and diversifying your portfolio. If you were investing in stocks and had to diversify, you would have to select at least 10 stocks carefully from different sectors. This can be a lengthy, time-consuming process.

☐ **Cost Efficient:**

We all know that when you buy in bulk, the cost per unit reduces drastically. This is known as economies of scale. A mutual fund scheme has lakhs of investors. Hence, they can achieve huge economies of scale. This reduces the fund's overall expenses. Similarly, other expenses are shared among all unitholders. So, the expense per unitholder also reduces. When expenses reduce, the returns earned by investors increase. Hence, mutual funds are one of the most cost-efficient investment options in India. Passively managed mutual funds like Index funds carry a lower expense ratio and are highly cost-efficient.

☐ Professional Portfolio Management:

Mutual fund schemes are professionally managed by fund managers. These fund managers are financial experts with years of stock market experience. Fund managers do in-depth research on stocks before taking any investment decision. They also constantly monitor the portfolio to ensure optimal returns. Historically, actively managed mutual funds have generated superior returns than passively managed funds.

☐ Diversification:

Diversification is the biggest advantage of mutual funds. When you invest in mutual funds, your investment is divided and invested into various stocks. By doing this, the overall risk of the fund reduces. Diversification also increases your chances of earning higher returns as you get to participate in the growth of all top stocks.

☐ Easy purchase and redemption:

Mutual fund schemes are sold through various channels. Most banks, broking houses, wealth management companies, and fintech companies offer online and offline transaction facilities. Many apps facilitate mutual fund transactions, as well. All this makes investing in mutual funds very convenient. Compare schemes, start an investment, redeem units—you can do everything from the comfort of your home.

☐ Tax-saving benefits:

Some mutual fund schemes offer tax benefits under Section 80C of the Income Tax Act. Equity-Linked Savings Schemes (ELSS), for example, is also known as tax-saver funds. They come with good returns as well as tax benefits under section 80C (it differs from country to country)

☐ Flexibility to switch:

You can freely switch from one scheme to another scheme of the same mutual fund house. Maybe the equity market is overheated, and you want to keep your money safe. You could move your investment from an equity scheme to a debt fund offered by the same AMC.

☐ **Liquidity: -**

Closed-ended funds have their units listed at the stock's exchanges, thus they can be bought and sold at their market values. Over and above this the units can be directly redeemed to the mutual funds as and when they announce the repurchase

☐ **Choice: -**

A large amount of mutual funds offers the investor a wide variety to choose from. An investor can pick up a scheme depending on his risk/ return profile.

RISK OF MUTUAL FUNDS

Mutual Funds may face the following risks, leading to non-satisfactory performance.

1. **Standard Risks**: -

Mutual Fund and securities investments are subject to investment risks such as trading volumes, settlement risks, liquidity risks, and default risks including the possible loss of principal. And there is no assurance or guarantee that the objective of the mutual fund scheme will be achieved.

2. **Scheme-Specific Risks: -**

The level of risk in mutual funds depends on the types and objectives of the mutual fund's scheme. Equity mutual funds schemes are riskier as compared to balance mutual funds schemes.

1) **Schemes Investing in Equity:** - Describes briefly risks associated with an   investment in equity.

2) **Schemes Investing in Bonds: -**   Describes briefly risks associated with fixed incomes products like credit risk, prepayment risk, liquidity risk, etc.

3) **Risks Associated with Investing in Securitized Debt:** - if the scheme invests in these instruments.

4) **Risks associated with Investing in Derivatives:** - if the scheme invests in these instruments.

5) **Schemes investing in Foreign Securities:** - Describes briefly risks associated with investing in the foreign market.

6) **Fund Manager Failure risks:** - Mutual fund unit investors face the risk of the fund manager not performing.

7) **Interest Rates Risks, Valuations Risks: -** Investment in mutual funds units involves interest rates and valuation risks.

3. Other risks involved in mutual funds: -

☐ Past performance of the AMC does not guarantee the future performance of the schemes.

☐ Excessive diversification of portfolio, losing focus on the securities of the key segments.

☐ Too much concentration on large-cap or blue-chip stocks which are high priced, and which do not offer more than average return

☐ Fund managers being unaccountable for the poor performance of funds.

☐ Failure to identify the risk of the schemes as distinct from the risk of the market.

☐ Unresearched forecast on income, profits, and government policies.

☐ Many mutual funds may provide positive returns, but many provide returns   less than the benchmarks.

☐ Under Performances in comparison to peers.

DISADVANTAGES OF MUTUAL FUNDS

1. **Cost despite negative returns: -**

    Investors must pay sales charges, annual fees, and other expenses regardless of how the fund performs, even if the fund went on to perform poorly.

2. **Lack OF Control: -**

    Investors typically cannot ascertain the exact make-up of the fund's portfolio at any given time nor can they directly influence which securities the fund manager buys and sells or the timing of those trades.

3. **Price Uncertainty: -**

    With an individual's stocks, investors can obtain real-time or close to real-time pricing information with relative ease by checking financial websites or by calling their broker. Investors can also monitor how a stock's prices at which investors purchase or redeem units will typically depend on the fund's NAV which the fund might not calculate until many hours after investors have placed their order.

Chapter - 4

story

Story for financial freedom to pursue passion

"Wow!" Luci

exclaimed for the nth time as she gaped at the singing by the celebrity singer, Christina.

Luci had always wanted to sing. She had spent innumerable evenings singing and learning signing instruments in her childhood. However, as she grew up, her parents decided that she must study architecture as it was tough to make a living as a singer. Luci was good in studies, especially maths and physics, but her real interest lay in singing. Nonetheless, Luci was aware of the hardships struggling singers have to endure to make a living in the initial year of their careers, and she didn't want any of it.

Growing up in a middle-class household, Luci had always wanted to earn enough money to buy the things she had always wanted, from dresses to shoes to expensive phones and much more!

A bright student, Luci bagged a well-paying job in a converted MNC that visited her college for placements. Almost a year in her new job, Luci is living nothing short of a dream. She earns well, and most will say, lives well. Her wardrobe boasts of the top labels and her apartment is a swanky new car.

That Sunday morning, with nothing much to do, Luci spotted a little advert announcing the **'singing concert'** being held not far from her apartment. Luci had heard about the famous singer Christina, and out of a whim, she made plans to attend the workshops.

Luci 's childhood aspirations of becoming a singer once again surface. In a short while, Christina had sung a very popular song to the audios.

During the break, Luci walked over to Christina and asked a lot of questions about singing. She also confessed how she always wanted to become a singer, but following her parents' advice, she became an architect instead.

"May I ask you a personal question, Christina?" Luci asked hesitantly. "Now that you have become famous, is it easier to earn more money by selling your album?" do you still depend on the album and concert to pay your bills? Please don't mind my questions, I know I am being rude, but I need to find an answer because I want to follow your footsteps and become a full-time singer," Luci blurted out in a single breath, fearing a rebuke from Christina.

But Christina found the young girl's curiosity to be amusing. She had a good heart laugh before saying, "oh my god, Luci! Don't worry. Meet me after the concert, and I will tell you my financial secrets," Christina finished her sentence with a conspiring wink, and Luci walked back to her seat in half excitement and half embarrassment.

After the concert, Christina and Luci planned to sit in a café to chat.

"But before we get there, we need to stop at a nearby place," announced Christina.

After a few minutes" the driver, Christina parked her car in front of an old, sprawling building. 'Children of God' was printed on a blue board at the entrance of the building.

"Wanna come along?" Christina asked Luci, who readily jumped out of the car.

It is hard to say if Luci was more shocked or confused when she saw Christina handing over the cheque from the concert to the sister at the orphanage. Peering over Christina's shoulders, Luci saw that it was the same cheque that the concert owner had given Christina after the concert. The cheque bore the same name she read on the board at the entrance of the building- 'children of the god charitable trust.' But that was not all, Christina took out a few more fat cheques, had handed them over to the sister with a warm smile.

As they drove to the café, Luci's head was bursting with questions.

'If she donates her hard-earned money, how does she survive?'

'Is she an heiress to a large business empire?'

'Is she too gullible to give away her earring to charity without keeping anything for herself?'

Luci bombarded Christina with all the questions that were raging in her mind. After listening to Luci's question, Christina said, "Yes, I give away all the money that I earn from the concert and album to various charities." This is because they need that money more than I do. And no, I don't come from a rich family. My father worked in a mid-level government job.

Christina revealed to Luci that she always wanted to make the world beautiful with singing and kindness. On her 15th birthday. She met a distant uncle who was very successful and quite wealthy. It was he who gave Christina the mantra of 'financial independence retire early.

Christina also revealed that, like Luci, her parents, too, wanted her to pursue a professional degree to support herself financially. So, Christina did her MBA from a good business school and landed a challenging yet well-paying job. She made it a point to invest as much as she could from each month's salary.

"I realised my financial goals before I turned 30, and by 35, my portfolio was earning more income each month than my salary! That was when I stopped working for money".

Christina told Luci that she and her husband both are financially independent before turning 40 years. "With our money making more money for us, we got free from the stress of earning to pay our expenses. My husband teaches English and maths to children in orphanages and slums, and I try to help NGOs and community initiatives with money earned from my album and concert," Christina said with calm contentment.

That Sunday, Luci's life changed for good. Christina happily agreed to mentor Luci in singing as well as in financial planning and investing. Luci is now on the road to creating a self-sustaining portfolio and retiring from her job, much before she turns 40!

Working to retire early

"Hey, Vishnu!" Clinton called from the water cooler where Sneha and Reshma were talking excitedly.

As Vishnu approached the exuberant group, Clinton patted his back in a friendly manner & asked, "so, you are coming to the club tonight, right?"

Vishnu smiled, and politely declined the offer.

"What, man! Today we are getting our first paycheque. We ought to celebrate!" said Reshma, who seemed incredulous at the idea of not parting when you have the money.

"Come on, brother. Don't be a scrooge, let's go and party, we deserve it after a month-long hard work," cajoled Clinton. But Vishnu was firm.

"I am not a miser, dear. I just want to manage my money responsibly so that when I need it, it's there for me."

"Oh, big words," Sneha pulled a face at Vishnu.

The group had been working together in the IT firm for the past year, but they had known each other for a good part of four years during their engineering program. All four had cracked the campus placement with a leading IT MNC and were now fortunate to be working together on the same project.

Vishnu was a smart, sensible, brooding young man who didn't act on impulse. He took his time to turn over things in his mind before deciding. Kind, mellow and soft-spoken, Vishnu was perhaps the only one in the group having a concrete vision of his future. And the beginning of all his dreams and ambition was to attain financial independence much earlier in his life.

Vishnu had always looked up to his cousin, Yash, who was a serial entrepreneur and deeply devoted to several social causes. Yash had attained financial independence in his early thirties and then on, he devoted his time, intellect, and efforts to initiatives and projects that were close to his heart.

Yash had taken his younger brother under his wings when he turned 15. Yash would spend a lot of time with Vishnu, explaining to him the nuances of wealth creation.

"Attaining financial freedom is the first, and the most definitive step towards growing rich," Yash had once shared with Vishnu.

Through Yash, Vishnu learned that by making small, yet regular investments for a long period of time can help anyone grow rich. Vishnu had taken the pledge to create a substantial corpus of money by the time he turned 40 years old.

When he finished telling his story to his friends and explained his commitment towards creating a self-sustaining portfolio over the next fifteen years, Vishnu asked his friends, "so, what do you suggest? Should I go out with guys and spend a major portion of my salary in one night," or should I invest the same money to attain financial independence?

"I think I agree with you Vishnu," it was Reshma who broke the silence. "But can you tell us more about the investment part? I mean, there are hundreds of investment options out there, and not all are safe or effective," she voiced her concerns.

"You can start investing in the equity market, which has given consistent returns over the years" provided you invest for a long time. A good way to invest in equities is via mutual funds through monthly payments. A mutual fund is managed by a qualified fund manager so that you don't have to worry about which stock to invest," said Vishnu. "The compounding effect in mutual funds investment pays rich returns, and only by exercising sheer determination, and financial discipline, can you attain financial independence. I suggest you guys must invest at least 25% of your salary," he added.

"Well, you are saying this word, financial independence, over and over again. What does it mean? Asked a clueless Sneha."

Vishnu explained to her that financial independence meant, "not having to work to pay your bills."

As a perplexed group of young engineers looked on, Vishnu urged them to imagine a life where they don't have to slog every day just to earn enough money to pay the bill. Instead, hobbies, or passion without having to worry about paying the expenses.

"Once your portfolio grows significantly, it starts earning sizable returns, even when you stop investing. Hobbies, or passion without having to worry about paying the expenses."

The new insights dawned upon the group, and they started to see a lot of sense in Vishnu's attitude toward spending money.

"I know what you say is cent percent correct, Vishnu. But I really wanted to let my hair down and have a good time," said Clinton gloomily.

But Reshma cheered him up instantly. "We can still have a lot of fun! Let's meet at Vishnu's apartment this evening, split the cost for food and beverages, play some games and sing songs," she said excitedly.

Clinton liked the idea much. "I will get my guitar and Sneha can sing. We will have our own little party of friends!" he exclaimed.

The friend high-fives just before being shooed away to their workstations by their project manager who hated youngsters wasting time near the water cooler.

The wealthy peon

Sunil was merely 16 years old when Mr. Robert found him outside his office building, pleading with the security personnel for work. Mr. Robert took an instant liking to the boy, who, in spite of his impoverished circumstances, had the self-respect to deny an offer of money.

"I don't beg to take charities, sir. I have studied till the 10th standard. If you give me a job, I will work hard and be forever loyal to you."

Sunil's job was easy. He had to make tea and serve it with biscuits twice during the day to the small team of investors working in Mr. Robert's financial consulting firm. Yes, Peter got the opportunity to work at a place where everyone spoke equity markets and stocks and bulls and bears. Besides serving tea, Peter volunteered to do fieldwork too, learning a great deal about investment vehicles, financial institutions and agencies.

Right from his initial day at the office, Mr. Robert encourages Peter to invest in the USA growth story. He showed him statistics, charts and figures revealing the growth in the Indian equity market.

"Peter, the share market is the best place to invest, however, you need not sell your shares too early. Those who remain investment in the equity market for long are the only ones who make real wealth"

He also told Peter that those who neither have large sums to invest nor the knowledge to pick the right stock must invest in equity through mutual funds. Though he earned a small income, Peter managed to invest little each month in a mutual fund through SIP.

Honest, hardworking and intelligent, Peter made quick progress at work, becoming an experienced field boy in a couple of years. However, he insisted that he would continue serving tea to the staff, which he considered as his family members. Years passed, and Peter continued to work at the office, gaining more financial knowledge each year. He was also investing around 30% of his salary in his portfolio, which was growing at a phenomenal rate.

During this while, a few kind and intelligent team members motivated and guided Peter to study further. With their teaching and mentoring, Peter completed his post graduation through correspondence courses. He also surprised everyone in the office, including Mr. Robert, by securing key financial certifications.

It was Peter's 40th birthday, and everyone at the office had gathered in the lobby to celebrate. Mr. Robert and the entire staff had planned a surprise gift for him. Mr. Robert, unbeknownst to Peter, had also invited his wife and ten-year- old son to office.

"Before you cut the cake, we have a surprise for you," announced Mr. Robert.

Peter was pleasantly surprised to see his family. He let his son blow out the candles and cut cake with him.

After refreshment, Mr. Robert made another announcement, "dear peter it is time for your second surprise for the day," he paused for dramatic effect, "from today onwards, you are promoted as a financial consultant at our firm." The office lobby erupted with applause and cheers.

Peter was overwhelmed with emotions. He hugged Mr. Robert and fighting the tears of joy, and tremor in his voice, spoke, "I don't know how to thank you all for this great honour. Without the love, help and warmth given by all of you and Robert sir, I may have lost my way in this world. All of you are worthy of my worship…"

Peter took time to recover from his breakdown, while his wife and Mr. Robert soothed him.

"I know that you all love me and want me to succeed in life. This I will never forget. However, I can't take up this new title,"Peter looked around to see a stunned audience.

"In fact, I would not be able to work at this office anymore, at least not full time," he added.

Everyone in the office had a quizzical look on their faces. To end the confusion, Peter spoke again, "my dear friends, thanks to you all that I have learnt some very important lessons in life. You all taught me the important of compassion, caring, education, and above all, financial independence"

"Robert sir encouraged me to start investing as soon as I got my first salary," Peter smiled warmly, looking loving at his boss.

"Over the years, I have been able to build a large, self-sustaining portfolio, where my returns exceed much more than my humble needs. I don't need to work for money anymore."

As the crowd smiled appreciatively, Mr. Robert patted Peter back, much like a pound teacher presenting his prodigy to the world.

"Coming up from the dark abyss of poverty, I know there are countless more who are enslaved by money, and without any scope of education, will probably never be able to provide the basic comforts of their families. I wish to use my money to provide a dignified life to people living below the poverty line. It is my dream to skill the poor, preparing them for job opportunities. Additionally, I also wish to offer financially disciplined, and eventually, financially independent."

The lobby once again erupted in loud cheering, hearing Peter's noble plan. Mr. Robert raised his hand to restore silence in the office, and taking Peter's arm, he said, "dear colleagues and friends! Today Peter has proved that he is not only a bright investor but also a great human being. I commit to supporting him in his social work fully and would invite all of you to help him make a great change in society." Mr. Robert's word was received with sincere enthusiasm from the entire staff.

And that's how the wealthy peon embarked on a journey to help the poor see the path to wealth creation.

Working to retire early Working to retire early Working to retire early.

Chapter - 5

MMS technique

Now many of you have asked the question, what is that MMS technique?

So, the MMS technique is none other than a **money management system** that helps many people to save money after getting their salary.

Many people complained that I don't save money at the end of the money. All my money is spent on day-to-day expenses. Many of you try that at the end of the month I save several money, but they fail.

Now you think that yah, the same problem I face in my life but I can't get the solution. So don't worry, in this book I will give you a very interesting technique that you will imply In your life.

Before we start to learn the MMS technique there are the four types of people surrounding us.

The first type of people is spenders. This type of person spends their money on unnecessary things. Like they go shopping every week, and every weekend they are going to watch a movie and have fun, they have unnecessary products like status that they don't require or shoes, or clothes they actually don't require but they purchase.

This is the first type of people and now the second type of people is the saver.

Those people who save a little bit of their income at the end of the month. But the problem starts when they have to use their hard earned saving income in any emergency case. People lose all their savings in medical emergencies. So that is also not a good way to save money.

The third type of person is a Holder. These types of people hold their money in their homes or in the bank. His money is not growing in the future, the value of that money is deprecated year by year. This type of feeling that my money is not safe was accepted by me.

And the fourth and last type of people is none-other than MONK. They live their life without tension. They don't have to think about how to earn money and where to spend money. They live their life happily and by meditation they live a peaceful life.

So here we see that there are four types of people surrounding us, now you have to decide what kind of people you are.

Finally, we can learn the money management system to earn more money and live your life financially free after a certain age that you have retired.

So here in this technique, there is a seven jar. In that jar, you must distribute your monthly income according to the MMS technique.

1. Freedom - 10%

2. Health – 10%

3. Spending -10%

4. Necessities – 50%

5. Learning – 10%

6. Entertainment – 5%

7. Contribution – 5%

All these seven techniques we learn one by one but after learning this technique you have to set with pen and paper and distribute your monthly money according to these seven techniques. And tell your family, this is our monthly budget. That we spend accordingly.

1. Freedom fund

Freedom fund now many people think that what is the freedom fund? What I have to do is fund freedom funds. Here my friend's freedom fund is the fund that helps you to become financially free. Here you have to invest at least 10% of your income in the freedom fund. Here "you are not working for money, money works for you" now you are thinking how it could be possible that money works for us. Yes, it is possible that.

You have saved some part of your monthly income. And that saved money to invest in a mutual fund, stock, bonds, debentures etc.

Now you have a question how much money I should invest? and the answer is it's totally according to you 10%, 15%, 20%. But if you invest more money like vies you started investing 20% of your salary at the age of 20 then you know what the result is. You are playing in crore at the age of 40 to 45.

How many people don't have a pension? If sometimes they see their investment is negative. They panic and withdraw all their investment and savings. You don't have to do that. I saw many youngsters start a mutual fund at the age of 20. But they don't have pensions. And close their mutual fund account and they are under 90% of the world population.

The fact is only 1% of people live a standard life and 9% of people live a comfortable life and the rest 90% of people have struggled their whole life.

Now you have to decide if you want to count yourself in 1% or in 90% of the world population.

Now I share with you a very beautiful story of the financial freedom story of Mr. Gujju.

Mr. Gujju is a small and famous actor in Gujarat. His company Gujju enterprise performs very well and grows every year.

One day he decides to retire at the age of 50. And the next morning he call his family member in the hall and distributed his wealth. The house on his son's name, and the bank FD on his daughter's name. Now he has only a gold chain. That he gifted to his beautiful wife.

One year later his son was bored by his parents and threw them on a road side. They both decided to go to his daughter's home but after a 2 month daughter blamed his father for the robbery of 5 lakh rupees.

And Mr. Gujju and his wife left that home also and went to his village side. Now Mr. Gujju starts labour work to fulfil their need. But after a week his wife is ill and doesn't have money for his treatment and she dies.

So what we learn from this story is Mr. Gujju is well stable in his life but he makes one mistake and that is he transfers all his wealth to his son and daughter before he dies and the result is he has to start his life from the very first step. He is able to live his life very beautifully after his retirement but he can't. So live your retirement enjoyable, plan properly your retirement. Never ever transfer your wealth to your children before you die.

2. Emergency Fund

The second jar is an emergency jar. In this second jar you have to put 10% of your salary in the emergency fund jar. This fund will be use in any medical emergency or challenges, or any problems

We all see the corona pandemic. We can't predict that we have to sit 3-4 months at least in your house, we have to lockdown ourselves. At that time 90% of people don't have any emergency money that they could use during pandemic. Many people don't have to money to pay this medical expenses. At that time this emergency fund jar help you a lots.

Not every medical emergency people have to face but you also face many challenges like losing a job or shutting your business. At that time you have at least that much money that you can spend at least for six months.

Not every time medical emergency people have to face but you also face many challenges like job loose or shutdown your business at that time you have at least that much money that you can spend that at least for six months

This is the situation where you use an emergency fund jar. I saw many people that have such a type of emergency fund and they use it during a corona pandemic.

3. Spending Fund

The third jar is the spending jar. Now you think that spending a jar means I have to fulfil all my needs from this jar.

Before you think I'm some crazy disciplined saver, let me give you some room to breathe and relax. 10% of your income is going to go to having as much fun as you want.

So the answer is no. You don't have to fulfil your needs from this jar but things you have to buy from that are not necessary in your life like TV, fridge, washing machine, or fast food, travelling, etc. It means all the expenses that entertain you.

This spending fund jar is also known as an entertainment jar also.

According to the research an average person spends 30% of their salary on desires and wants and dining out.

Many experts say that people have to control their needs to implement some simple things into your life by decreasing your daily needs make budgets. Have control on your desire.

I suggest that if you have a usage burden of debt then don't create an entertainment jar account. First focus on how to reduce the debt.

Here there is a twist. The twist is you have to empty this jar to avoid overspending or under-spending, make sure you use up the money from this jar at least every few months. This allows you to spend without guilt, and to also gradually improve your standard of living as your income increases.

4. Necessities/ Needs

The fourth jar in this money management system is a Necessity. Necessities or Needs take 50 percent of your total income.

Now the question is what do I consider in my need? Now the answer is Housing expenses, Grocery, Transportation,

Medical, Rent, Bills. This all things are considered under the Needs.

What types of bills should be considered. Bills that you pay every month or every 3 months. That should be considered for example – phone bills, light bills, water bills.

You have to maintain all of your needs under 50 per-cent of your income during your whole life. If it is more than 50 per-cent then you have to give attention to that necessitie fund department. You have to reduce 50 per-cent to your all needs or necessities.

The percentage of your necessities fund will be reduced over the period And that reduces the amount you have to put in the investment jar or a freedom fund for the upliftment of your life.

Let's understand by a simple story. Mr. Jack has a salary of rupees 1 lakh per month.

Then he follows the 7-jar system in his life accordingly in his necessities jar 50 percent of his income means he puts in 50000 per month. Now over the years he decreased the percentage of necessities funds. After 10 years, his needs are 40% of his income and the 10% remaining amount he transfers into freedom funds.

5. Learning

Did you think that people have to continue their learning until their last breath? I totally agree with you if your answer is "yes".

If anyone tells you that I stop learning after the age of 23. Then he is telling a lie because we learn that people continue their learning until his last breath. It doesn't matter whether you study in school or in college. Many times life gives us a big problem that we never face in our life. But still we find solutions anyhow and many times we can't find the solution.

At that time, we need a guru. That he or she helped us to come out from that problem. Sometimes they charge or may not charge money. If we talk about the business at times also we need a guru to grow business and to find and solve that problem that we cant see.

For that reason, we have required a learning fund and a learning fund requires 10% of your monthly income. I saw many people who make a learning fund but never use it. He never upgrades himself. And that money transfers into an entertainment fund. So, you don't have to make this type of silly mistake. Such times many trainers come to your city to attend his seminar or workshop to upgrade yourself.

Even I attain 5-6 seminars and workshops during the year to upgrade myself and to live a better life. Today I wrote the book at the age of 20 because I upgraded and learned how to earn money to become an author and I know how to manage money.

So here I share with you a beautiful story of Kashyap from Pune, Maharashtra.

This guy takes 15 tablets every day. He has been depressed for the last 7 years. One day he knows that one amazing trainer will come to his city. go there to attain the workshop. At that time his salary was 15000 per month. He has to manage all of his income in 15000 only. That time he attained the workshop of Rs 8000. During the break, he got a chance to meet the trainer and tell his problem. The trainer decided to help him to come out from depression free of cost. Now Kashyap is the owner of 7 different businesses and he and his family are so happy to see Kashyap in a positive mindset.

That's why I tell you to create a learning fund. I won't tell you that you also have a similar type of problem, but this seminar helps a lot of people.

6. Entertainment fund

The second last fund is entertainment funds. This fund contains 5% of your monthly income.

Now in the entertainment fund what you have to do is the money that you spend behind the movies and for tourism that you have to manage from the entertainment fund.

According to the spending jar you have to finish all money from this fund.

Even in this jar you also have to transfer all money into your investment jar or in a freedom jar but it is compulsory to do this.

Your family has 5 members out of which there are 3 earning members so it is not compulsory to create different entertainment accounts but even 3 members also contribute their 5 percent income combined.

I think we don't have to discuss more about this fund because you people are very smart about what my audience is, and you know what things are under the entertainment fund or what not.

7. Contributions Fund

This is the last jar of our MMS techniques and that is the contribution fund.

At least 5 percent of your income is a contribution to society. Now you have several questions: where to contribute, how to contribute?

The answer is very simple in the contribution fund money you can contribute to old age homes, children who have no parents I mean (orphaned) children, or those people who don't get food for all three times, in winter season many people who sleep on the footpath that people you can give a blanket, those children those who have no money to study even that is also a contribution to society. Take care of animals and birds; they cannot speak like us.

There are some examples of how people can contribute to society. I saw many people that contribute 15 to 30 percent of his income.

Chapter - 6

Is Something Better Than a Mutual Fund?

Now you people think that we learn all about the mutual fund, how it is better for us, how its give benefit in long team RIGHT? And now I say that something that is more profitable then mutual fund. I beat you that this thing will give more profit as compare to mutual fund in long-team with very less expenses.

Are you excited to know about that ? there is the answer

EXCHANGE TRADED FUND

Yes, the **Exchange Traded Fund (ETF)** will give more profit than mutual funds. Very few investors know about the ETF because no more people have knowledge about ETF.

So I will explain the whole concept of an ETF in this book.

WHAT IS an ETF?

So, what exactly are ETFs? Think of them as a convenient investment vehicle that combines the best features of both stocks and mutual funds. They are like a basket filled with a variety of stocks, bonds, or other assets that you can buy or sell on the stock exchange, just like a regular stock.

One of the coolest things about ETFs is that they provide you with a way to own a diverse portfolio without having to pick and choose individual stocks yourself. You get instant exposure to a wide range of companies or sectors, helping you spread out your risk and potentially increase your chances of success.

ETFs are designed to be flexible and cost-effective. You can buy or sell them throughout the trading day, just like any other stock. This means you have the freedom to jump in or out of the market whenever you want, giving you more control over your investments.

Another great aspect of ETFs is their transparency. The underlying holdings of an ETF are usually disclosed on a daily basis, allowing you to know exactly what you own. This transparency gives you a clear picture of where your money is being invested and allows you to make informed decisions.

What's even better is that ETFs come in a variety of flavours to suit different investment goals and preferences. Whether you're interested in broad market exposure, specific sectors, or even niche themes like renewable energy or artificial intelligence, there's likely an ETF out there that matches your interests.

Now, it's important to remember that investing always carries some degree of risk, and ETFs are no exception. The value of your investment can fluctuate based on the performance of the underlying assets. But by doing your research, diversifying your holdings, and aligning your investments with your financial goals, you can mitigate some of those risks.

So, whether you're a seasoned investor or just starting out, ETFs can be a fantastic tool to help you build a well-rounded investment portfolio. They offer simplicity, flexibility, and the potential for long-term growth.

Remember, though, we're just scratching the surface here. If you're interested in exploring ETFs further, it's always a good idea to consult with a financial advisor or do some additional research to find the ETFs that best align with your investment objectives.

Types Of ETF

1. Broad Market ETFs:

These ETFs aim to replicate the performance of a broad market index, such as the S&P 500, Nifty-50 or the total stock market. They provide exposure to a wide range of companies across different sectors and are great for investors seeking diversification and overall market returns.

2. Sector ETFs:

If you're interested in specific industries or sectors, sector ETFs are here to fulfil your curiosity. They focus on a particular sector, such as technology, healthcare, or energy. These ETFs allow you to invest in companies within a specific industry and capitalise on their growth potential.

3. Bond ETFs:

Bond ETFs provide exposure to fixed-income securities like government bonds, corporate bonds, or municipal bonds. They are popular among income-oriented investors looking for stable returns and potentially lower risk compared to stocks. Bond ETFs come in different durations, credit qualities, and yield preferences to cater to various investment strategies.

4. International ETFs:

Are you eager to expand your investment horizons beyond your home country? International ETFs allow you to invest in companies from different countries and regions worldwide. These ETFs offer exposure to international markets and can be a great way to diversify your portfolio globally.

5. Commodity ETFs:

If you're interested in investing in commodities like gold, silver, oil, or agricultural products, commodity ETFs are a convenient option. They can track the performance of a specific commodity or a basket of commodities, providing exposure to their price movements without the need for physical ownership.

6. Currency ETFs:

Currency ETFs allow you to invest in foreign currencies. They track the Exchange rates between different currencies and can be used as a tool for hedging currency risk or speculating on currency movements. Currency ETFs are a way to diversify your investment beyond stocks and bonds.

7. Dividend ETFs:

Dividend ETFs focus on companies that regularly pay dividends. These ETFs aim to provide investors with a steady income stream through dividends while also potentially benefiting from capital appreciation. They can be an attractive option for

investors seeking both income and growth.

8. Smart Beta ETFs:

Smart Beta ETFs incorporate an additional layer of strategy by applying alternative index-weighting methodologies. These methodologies can include factors like low volatility, value, momentum, or quality. Smart Beta ETFs seek to outperform traditional market-weighted ETFs by targeting specific investment factors.

9. Thematic ETFs:

Thematic ETFs revolve around specific investment themes or trends, such as renewable energy, artificial intelligence, cybersecurity, or robotics. They allow investors to align their portfolios with their personal interests or beliefs while potentially capitalising on emerging trends and industries.

10. **Active ETFs:**

While most ETFs are passively managed, actively managed ETFs have a team of portfolio managers who actively make investment decisions. They aim to outperform a specific benchmark or index by actively selecting securities. Active ETFs combine the benefits of ETFs, such as transparency and intraday trading, with the expertise of active management.

Remember, each type of ETF comes with its own set of characteristics and risk factors. It's essential to thoroughly research and understand the specifics of each ETF before investing. Consulting with a financial advisor can also provide valuable insights tailored to your investment goals.

Now you have a better understanding of the different types of ETFs available. So go ahead and explore the world of ETFs, find the ones that align with your investment strategy, and embark on your journey towards financial success!

HOW TO BUY ETFS

Buying ETFs is a straightforward process, and here's a friendly step-by-step guide to help you get started:

1. Determine your investment goals: Before diving into buying ETFs, it's crucial to establish your investment objectives. Are you looking for long-term growth, income, or diversification? Clarifying your goals will help you select the most suitable ETFs for your needs.

2. Research and select ETFs: Conduct thorough research on the different ETFs available in the market. Consider factors such as the ETF's investment strategy, expense ratio, performance history, holdings, and the index it aims to track. Look for ETFs that align with your investment goals and risk tolerance.

3. Choose a brokerage account: To buy and sell ETFs, you'll need to open an account with a brokerage firm. Look for a reputable brokerage that offers access to a wide range of ETFs, has user-friendly trading platforms, and provides excellent

customer service. Compare fees, commissions, and any account minimums that may apply.

4. Fund your brokerage account: Once you've chosen a brokerage, you'll need to fund your account. This usually involves transferring funds from your bank account to your brokerage account. Follow the instructions provided by your chosen brokerage to complete this process.

5. Place your ETF order: Log into your brokerage account and navigate to the trading platform. Search for the specific ETF you want to buy by its ticker symbol or name. Enter the number of shares you wish to purchase and select the order type (market order or limit order). Review your order details and submit the trade.

6. Monitor your ETF investments: After buying ETFs, it's essential to keep an eye on your investments. Monitor the performance of your ETFs, review any news or updates related to the underlying assets or the ETF itself, and periodically reassess your investment strategy. This will help you stay informed and make any necessary adjustments to your portfolio.

Remember, investing in ETFs carries risks, including the potential loss of your investment. It's crucial to diversify your investments, conduct thorough research, and consider your risk tolerance before making any investment decisions. If you're unsure about the process or need assistance, don't hesitate to consult with a financial advisor who can provide personalised guidance.

Happy investing and may your ETF journey be filled with success and financial growth!

How i buy ETF

It's a very interesting way to buy ETF shares.

I buy shares when the price of shares are drop by 1% or more than 1%. I add a few ETF shares at the time of market down in my portfolio.

The effect is prices of ETFs will increase and my average cost is decrease. So I get more return on ETFs.

I buy MON-100, it's a share of American top-100 companies. Now I have 30 units of ETF and my return is more than 25% in just 6 months.

It's not a suggestion that you only have to buy this ETF you can also buy the share of Indian top 50 companies.

COMPARE MUTUAL FUND, INDEX FUND & ETFS

Now we are going to compare these 3 funds and analyse which one is better for our portfolio.

1. Expenses ratio. (Annual Commission)

    a. Mutual fund -- 0.5% to 2%

    b. Index fund -- 0.2% or Lesser

    c. ETF – 0.05%

2. Exit load.

    a. Mutual fund – 1%

    b. Index fund – NO

    c. ETF – NO

3. Tax.

    a. Mutual fund – Same in all

    b. Index fund – Same in all

    c. ETF – Same in all

4. Brokerage.

    a. Mutual fund – Yes

    b. Index fund – Yes

    c. ETF – No

5. Principal loss probabilities

    a. Mutual fund – Yes

    b. Index fund – Yes

    c. ETF – No

6. Company delisted OR Bankruptcy Risk

    a. Mutual fund – Yes

    b. Index fund – Yes

    c. ETF – No

7. Buy of NAV

    a. Mutual fund – End of Day

    b. Index Fund – End of Day

    c. ETF – Instant During Market Open

8. Can Trade

    a. Mutual fund – No

    b. Index fund – No

    c. ETF – Yes

9. Easy Selection

    a. Mutual fund – No

    b. Index fund – No

    c. ETF -- Yes

Chapter - 7

CREDIT CARD

It is very important that now is the time to get knowledge about the credit card in this decade. Because the demand for credit cards is increasing rapidly in INDIA. In India very few percent of people have required financial knowledge.

Now people think that's why I added this topic in this book. Right because its a essential need of our life in future. So we have to learn more about the credit card uses, benefits, drawbacks, how its impact on personal finance, which credit card is best for us, how we can manage that for better financial health.

A credit card is like having a convenient and flexible financial tool in your pocket! It's a little piece of plastic (or sometimes digital) that allows you to make purchases without having to carry around a wad of cash. Think of it as a loan from the bank or credit card issuer that you can use to buy things now and pay for them later.

With a credit card, you can shop online, pay bills, dine out, book flights, and indulge in all sorts of fun activities. It's like having your own mini shopping assistant with you at all times!

One of the great things about credit cards is that they often come with perks and rewards. Depending on the type of card you have, you might earn points, cashback, or even travel miles every time you use it. It's like getting a little bonus for your everyday spending.

But remember, as awesome as credit cards can be, they also come with responsibilities. It's essential to use them wisely and within your means. Paying your credit card bills on time and in full is important to avoid extra charges and keep your credit score in good shape.

So, if you're looking for a convenient and secure way to make purchases, a credit card can be your trusty companion. Just remember to use it responsibly and enjoy the perks and benefits that come along with it!

HISTORY

So the credit card was first introduced in America in the early 20th century. Credit cards are firstly used by malls as department store cards to give credit to their customers. Then in the 1950 dinner card was introduced by Frank McNamara. Initially it was intended to be used in restaurants for their meal. Then in 1958 the first official credit cards were introduced by American express and banks for the purpose of travelling and entertainment expenses. And finally in the 1990's to 2000's chip cards were introduced by your Mastercard and Visa card. It helps in reducing the risk of frauds. So this is the history of Credit cards.

Types Of Credit Card's

We all know that credit cards exist in the world but most people don't know that there are many types of Credit cards and the uses of that card are also different. So I will tell you about the different types of Credit cards here.

1. Basic credit card
2. Travel credit card
3. Fuel credit card
4. Reward credit card
5. Cash back credit card
6. Entertainment credit card
7. Student credit card

8. Business credit card
9. Balance transfer credit card
10. Premium credit card
11. Kishan credit card

1. BASIC CREDIT CARD
- ☐ It is best for the first time user
- ☐ Regular features available
- ☐ Less credit limit
- ☐ Low interest charges
- ☐ Less annual maintenance fees

2. TRAVEL CREDIT CARD
- ☐ Domestic flight booking
- ☐ International flight booking
- ☐ Bus & railways ticket booking
- ☐ National & International hotel booking
- ☐ Airport lounge
- ☐ Air accident insurance
- ☐ Personal accident insurance
- ☐ Travel insurance
- ☐ Cab booking

3. FUEL CREDIT CARD
- ☐ Its give the amazing cashback
- ☐ Amazing reward

4. ENTERTAINMENT CREDIT CARD
- ☐ Movie ticket booking
- ☐ Resort booking
- ☐ Discount on movie ticket
- ☐ Free ticket some time

5. REWARD CREDIT CARD

- ☐ Its give additional reward point
- ☐ Interest rate higher then basic credit card

6. CASHBACK CREDIT CARD

- ☐ Its give only cashback on use of card

7. STUDENT CREDIT CARD

- ☐ It's only for full time course student
- ☐ Interest rate are very low than usual

8. BUSINESS CREDIT CARD

- ☐ It's only for businessman, professional
- ☐ Only for business use not for personnel use

9. BALANCE TRANSFER CREDIT CARD

- ☐ Some time people take credit from 2 or more cards and interest rate are high in some card at that time its help to transfer credit to one card to another

10. PREMIUM CARD

- ☐ This card is only for premium customer of bank

11. KISHAN CREDIT CARD

- ☐ Its gives low rate credit to the farmer

Drawbacks of Credit Cards

1. High-interest rates: Credit cards often come with high-interest rates, especially if you carry a balance from month to month. If you only make minimum payments, the interest charges can quickly add up, making it challenging to pay off the debt.

2. Debt accumulation: Credit cards make it easy to spend money that you may not have readily available. This can lead to impulsive purchases and overspending, resulting in accumulating debt. If you're not careful, credit card debt can become a burden and impact your financial well-being.

3. Fees: Credit cards may have various fees associated with them. These can include annual fees, balance transfer fees, cash advance fees, foreign transaction fees, and late payment fees. It's important to read the terms and conditions of your credit card to understand the fees involved.

4. Negative impact on credit score: Misusing or mishandling credit cards can negatively affect your credit score. Late payments, maxing out your credit limit, or applying for multiple credit cards within a short period can all have adverse effects on your creditworthiness.

5. The temptation to overspend: Credit cards provide easy access to credit, which can tempt individuals to spend beyond their means. Without proper budgeting and self-discipline, it's easy to

accumulate debt and find yourself in a financially challenging situation.

6. Security risks: Credit card fraud and identity theft are ongoing concerns in the digital age. Criminals can steal credit card information or make unauthorised charges, leaving cardholders vulnerable to financial loss and the hassle of resolving fraudulent activity.

7. Potential for financial dependency: Relying heavily on credit cards for everyday expenses can lead to a dependency on credit and an inability to live within your means. It's important to establish a balanced approach to credit card usage and maintain control over your finances.

To mitigate the drawbacks of credit cards, it's crucial to use them responsibly. Paying your credit card balance in full and on time, monitoring your spending, and keeping your credit utilisation low can help you avoid some of the pitfalls associated with credit card usage. Additionally, staying informed about your card's terms and conditions, practising financial discipline, and regularly reviewing your statements can contribute to a healthier financial relationship with credit cards.

Discipline way of use credit card

Now i share a beautiful story of Lily. She will teach us way of credit card use in life.

Once upon a time in the bustling city of Metropolis, there lived a young woman named Lily. Lily was a hardworking professional who had recently graduated from college and started her dream job at a marketing agency. Excited about her newfound independence, she decided it was time to apply for her first credit card.

Lily's motivation for getting a credit card was to establish a good credit history and take advantage of the various rewards and benefits that came with responsible credit card usage. She did her research, comparing different cards and their offerings, and finally settled on a card that provided cashback rewards and travel perks.

With her shiny new credit card in hand, Lily ventured into the world of financial responsibility. She vowed to use her card wisely, understanding that it was not free money but a tool that required careful management.

In the first few months, Lily made small purchases on her credit card, diligently paying off the balance in full each month. She kept track of her expenses, ensuring they aligned with her budget and her ability to pay them off promptly. Lily saw her credit score gradually improve, which brought her a sense of accomplishment and a boost of confidence in her financial journey.

One day, while browsing online, Lily stumbled upon a limited-time offer for a heavily discounted vacation package to a tropical paradise. The opportunity seemed too good to pass up, and Lily's heart yearned for a well-deserved getaway. Knowing she had saved up enough money to cover the cost, Lily made a well-informed decision to charge the travel expenses to her credit card.

The vacation was everything Lily had hoped for—relaxing, rejuvenating, and filled with beautiful memories. She savoured every moment, knowing she had made a wise financial decision by earning additional travel rewards through her credit card.

Upon returning from her trip, Lily was determined to pay off the vacation charges promptly. She devised a repayment plan and managed her finances diligently, making extra payments whenever possible. By sticking to her plan and remaining disciplined, she successfully cleared the balance within a few months, avoiding any interest charges.

Lily's responsible credit card usage didn't stop there. She continued to use her credit card for everyday purchases, strategically earning cash back rewards on groceries, gas, and other essentials. However, she never let the allure of rewards overshadow   her financial prudence. Lily maintained a monthly spending limit, ensuring that she never carried a balance beyond her means.

As time went on, Lily's responsible credit card usage and prompt payments were rewarded. Her credit score soared, allowing her to secure better interest rates for future endeavours like purchasing a car or even owning her own home.

Lily's success story with her credit card became an inspiration for her friends and colleagues. She shared her knowledge and experiences, emphasising the importance of responsible credit card usage, financial discipline, and the benefits it could bring.

In the end, Lily's credit card journey was not just about earning rewards or travelling to exotic destinations. It was about using the card as a tool for financial growth, responsible spending, and building a solid foundation for her future.

And so, Lily's story serves as a reminder that a credit card can be a valuable asset when used wisely, helping individuals achieve their dreams and navigate the world of personal finance with confidence and success.

How To Earn Money From Credit Cards

1. Reward earning

Let's understand this method by way of the story of Gemi.

Gemi goes shopping in a big mall in New York. It is the biggest mall in New York city. There she likes 2 dresses for $100. She takes out her credit card and swipes the card and $ 100 debit from his credit card. But the shopkeeper get $ 97 only. Now you have a question: gemi pays $100 but shopkeepers get only $97?

Because the credit card company cut 2-3% of the total amount from the shopkeeper. And that 2-3% money credit to your credit card. It depends on different companies. Now you can use those rewards for shopping and many other things. Sometimes companies give you cash back offers also.

Suppose Gemi has a cashback credit card then she gets $3 back to this account.this is the small amount $100. What if she spent $10,000 then Gemi got $300. If you use a credit card on a regular basis then at the end of year lots of money gets thought out.

You can spend on school fees, tuition fees, buying electric devices, for petrol, hotel rent, and so on. Did you imagine how much you have at the end of year?

2. No cost EMI

Every method we understand by the way of story. So under this method let's talk about lara.

Lara has a credit card from a visa company and his credit limit is $50,000. She can use $50,000 every month.

Lara has one son, his name is jack. And he is in school. Now Lara has to pay the fees of his son. So here Lara has two options. She can pay that fee from his debit or credit card.

She chose a credit card. She pays the $7,000 through credit card on EMI basis. Now she has to pay $1,000 every month to the credit card company. And the rest of the money is in the savings account of lara. Now she gets the benefit of interest from his bank. Suppose the interest rate is 4% then after 6 months she gets $140.

It's a small amount of $7,000. What if Lara spends $1,00,000 through a credit card. Then she gets $4,000 without doing anything. She can spend this $4,000 to buy an ETF then can you imagine how much she will have after 5-to-10 years.

Warning:- don't swipe credit card if the amount you swipe from credit card is not in your debit card otherwise you are in the trap of debt. Spend only the money that you have in your bank account through credit card.

3. Cashback Sip

In this method we took the story of Rohit. Rohit is an IT professional guy and he works with amazon. And his salary is 50,000 per month.

Rohit has a monthly fixed expense of 20,000. So this 20,000 he paid through credit card. You know I give a warning "spend only that money that you have in your bank account while you use your credit card".

So rohit did a fixed deposit of that 20,000 and he got 5% interest in auto convert fixed deposit account. So he gets 83 every month as an interest and rest and another monthly expense was 10,000 that also he pays through credit card. So another 45 he will get. In total he got 83+45 = 128. Rohit read our book so he got the knowledge of sip, mutual fund , and ETF, so he started investing in index mutual funds. Rohit starts sip of 1000 every month after the 10 year rohit monthly salary is 7,00,000 and his fixed expense is 2,30,000 and he follows this technique continuously. Now he gets fixed deposit interest of 770 every month and yearly 9,240 without doing anything and he is still doing sip 1000. So now in 10 years Rahul has 2,50,000 without doing anything and after 20 years it was 44,20,000.

This is assuming that Rahul invests only 1000 at a salary of 7,00,000. What if rahul increases it to 25,000 monthly index fund sip. It's in crores after 30 years.

About the Author

I was born in a middle class family. I see many ups and downs in these 20 years. When I get inspiration to write a book then I think of how to help those who struggle financially and many other usual issues in their life. So I wrote my first book SIP is F.I.R.E.

Instagram :- _dix_dhanani_

www.ingramcontent.com/pod-product-compliance
Lightning Source LLC
Chambersburg PA
CBHW022344290526
45786CB00014B/2424

Animal Peculiarity Volume 3 Part 1

By T.P Just

~~~

Copyright © 2010 by Terence Just. All rights reserved.

Get All The Books In The Series:

Animal Peculiarity Volume 1 [Part 1-8]
Animal Peculiarity Volume 2 [Part 1-8]
Animal Peculiarity Volume 3 [Part 1-8]
Just Enterprises

Table of Contents

1. Prologue
2. The Lion in old age
3. The Eagle's Feathers
4. The Crocodile and its young
5. The Moon, its influence on shellfish and Animals
6. The Basse and its otolith
7. The Elephant and its young
8. The Seal
9. The Malmignatte and the Asp, their bites
10. Frogs and their mating
11. The Snake and its eye-sight
12. The Halcyon and its nest
13. The Starfish and Oysters
14. The Fishing frog
15. Crayfish and Octopus
16. The Lion's tracks
17. The Argonaut
18. The 'Adonis' fish
19. Grafting of trees
20. The Sea-sheep and others
21. Insects, etc, born in plants
22. The Common Crab
23. The Sea-urchin
24. The largest of the Cetaceans